CARING ABOUT
YOUR WHOLE BODY

YOU SHOULD BE EATING

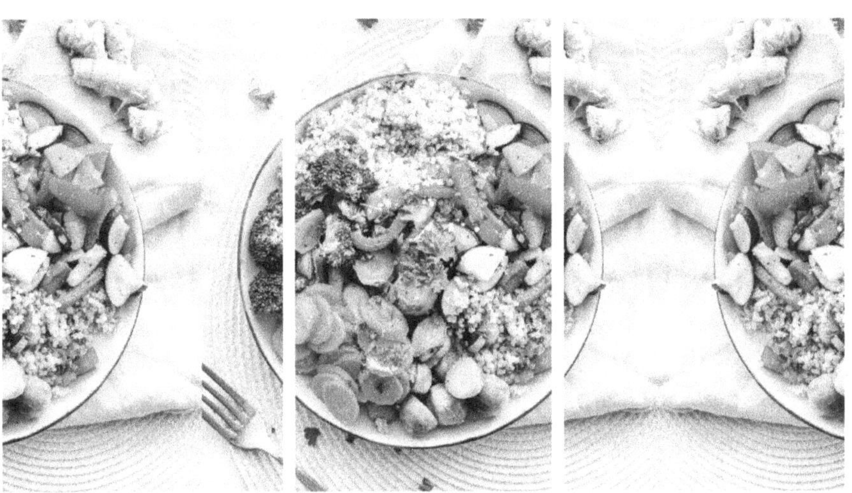

TO BEAT DISEASES

Health Writers

Copyright®2022 Health Writers

All Rights Reserved

MEDICAL DISCLAIMER

This book is created and published for informational purposes only. It is not intended to be a substitute for professional medical advice.

Always seek the guidance of your doctor or other qualified health professional with any questions you may have regarding your health or a medical condition. Never disregard the advice of a medical professional, or delay in seeking it.

TABLE OF CONTENT

HEALTHFUL EATING

SOME SUGGESTIONS FOR INCREASING YOUR DAILY INTAKE OF FRUITS AND VEGETABLES

LET'S TALK ABOUT DISEASES, VEGETABLES, AND FRUIT

IN ALFAFA, ARE RICH IN SPROUTS

ALFALFA SPROUTS NUTRITIONAL INFORMATION
ALFALFA SPROUTS OFFER A VARIETY OF BENEFICIAL PROPERTIES, INCLUDING THE FOLLOWING:
1. IT MAY AID IN THE BATTLE AGAINST CANCER
2. IT HAS THE POTENTIAL TO ASSIST YOU IN SHEDDING POUNDS
3. IT CAN AID IN THE TREATMENT OF TYPE 2 DIABETES
4. CHOLESTEROL LEVELS COULD BE REDUCED
5. IT MAY AID IN THE BATTLE AGAINST ILLNESSES IN YOUR BODY
6. IT MIGHT ASSIST WITH FOOD DIGESTIBILITY
7. IT HAS THE POTENTIAL TO ASSIST YOU IN GROWING AND RESTORING YOURSELF
8. IT HAS THE POTENTIAL TO HASTEN THE HEALING PROCESS

9. IT IS POSSIBLE TO AVOID OSTEOPOROSIS

10. IT HAS THE POTENTIAL TO INCREASE FAT BURNING

11. IT AIDS IN THE CARE OF ONE'S SKIN

WHY APPLES, EXACTLY

FIVE REASONS WHY APPLES ARE BENEFICIAL TO YOUR HEALTH

1. IT IS NUTRITIOUS

2. IT'S POSSIBLE THAT IT'LL ASSIST YOU IN LOSING WEIGHT

3. IT IS BENEFICIAL TO YOUR CARDIOVASCULAR SYSTEM

4. IT HAS BEEN RELATED TO A LOWER DIABETES RISK

5. IT MAY AID IN THE MAINTENANCE OF A HEALTHY DIGESTIVE SYSTEM

THERE IS SOMETHING ABOUT AVOCADOS

1. A LARGE NUMBER OF NUTRIENTS

2. GOOD FOR THE HEART

3. EXCELLENT FOR OBSERVING

4. IT MAY HELP PREVENT OSTEOPOROSIS

5. COMPONENTS MAY BE ABLE TO HALT THE PROGRESSION OF CANCER

BEET MAGIC

Here are several tempting ways to eat more beets, as well as five research-backed advantages of beets
1. Beet contains a high amount of nutrients while having a low-calorie count
2. They can aid in the reduction of excessive blood pressure, which is a major cause of heart disease
3. It can assist you in improving your athletic abilities
4. It has anti-inflammatory properties
5. May improve the health of your stomach

WHAT IS THE PURPOSE OF HEALTHY EATING?

1. The likelihood of developing cancer is reduced
3. Improving the health of one's intestines
4. The ability to remember information has improved
5. Preventing Weight Loss

CONCLUSION

HEALTHFUL EATING

Fruits and vegetables are beneficial to your health, but they are also beneficial to your weight. Fresh food has a lot of power, but not all fresh food is created equal.

Superfoods do include significantly more vitamins, minerals, and other nutrients than regular diets. By including these healthy ingredients in your diet, you may make your food more nutritious.

It can help lower blood pressure, cut the risk of heart disease and stroke, prevent some types of cancer, and maintain blood sugar levels, which can help keep hunger at bay. People who consume non-starchy fruits and vegetables such as apples, pears, and green leafy vegetables may be able to eat less. Their low glycemic indexes prevent blood sugar levels from rising, which may cause you to overeat.

There are at least nine major fruit and vegetable families, each with hundreds of different plant components that are beneficial to your health. Your body needs a variety of nutrients, so eat a variety of different types and colors of food. This guarantees that there are more beneficial plant chemicals present, as well as improving the appearance of the food.

Some suggestions for increasing your daily intake of fruits and vegetables

1. Place fruit in a visible location

Put some ready-to-eat washed whole fruits in a bowl, or slice colorful fruits and place them in a glass bowl in the fridge when you have a sweet tooth.

Browse the produce area for something fresh to try. Healthy food should contain a variety of ingredients and come in a variety of hues. On most days, at least one serving from each of the following groups should be consumed:

dark green leafy vegetables; yellow or orange fruits and vegetables; red fruits and vegetables; legumes (beans and peas); and citrus fruits.

2. Refrain from consuming the potatoes.

Choose vegetables with a variety of nutrients and easy-to-digest carbs.

3. Cook it

Cooking new vegetable-rich meals is a great way to expand your culinary horizons. Here are a few suggestions for increasing your vegetable intake: Salads, soups, and stir-fries are just a few examples of how you may incorporate more vegetables into your diet.

LET'S TALK ABOUT DISEASES, VEGETABLES, AND FRUIT

A diet high in fruits and vegetables can reduce the risk of heart disease and stroke, according to research.

Participants who ate more fruits and vegetables had a lower chance of dying from cardiovascular disease, according to a meta-analysis of studies that included 469,551 people. Each additional serving of fruits and vegetables reduced the death risk by 4%.

The Harvard-based nurses' health study and health professionals follow-up research included nearly 110,000 men and women, making it the largest and longest study to date. For 14 years, they were tracked.

Increasing your daily intake of fruits and vegetables lowers your risk of heart disease. People who ate more than 1.5 servings of fruits and vegetables per day were 30% less likely to suffer a heart attack or stroke.

Green leafy vegetables like lettuce, spinach, Swiss chard, and mustard greens were found to be the most significantly associated with a reduced risk of cardiovascular disease. This advantage came from all fruits and veggies, most likely. Broccoli, cauliflower, cabbage, and Brussels sprouts were also significant contributors. Oranges, lemons, limes, and grapefruit (together with their juice) played a significant role.

People who consumed more than 5 servings of fruits and vegetables per day had a 20% lower risk of coronary heart disease and stroke than those who consumed less than 3 servings per day. This was true for both heart attacks and strokes.

The Dietary Approaches to Stop Hypertension (DASH) study examined how a diet rich in fruits and vegetables, as well as low-fat dairy products, affects blood pressure. They also looked at how much saturated and total fat they ate. High blood pressure patients who followed this diet saw their blood pressure go down by about 11 mm Hg and their diastolic blood pressure (the lower number) go down by almost 6 mm Hg, which is as much as taking medicine can do.

People who took part in a study called the Optimal Macronutrient Intake Trial for Heart Health saw that this fruit and vegetable-heavy diet lowered blood pressure, even more, when some of the carbohydrates were replaced with healthy fat or protein.

People who ate a vegetarian diet had lower blood pressure, according to a meta-analysis of clinical trials and research published in 2014.

1. Cancer

Eating a lot of fruits and vegetables proved to protect against cancer in several early studies. Cohort studies, which follow large groups of healthy people for years and do not rely on information from the past, are more reliable than case-control studies. This is because cohort studies do not rely on prior data. Because there isn't a lot of evidence from cohort studies to support the notion that eating a lot of fruits and vegetables can prevent cancer.

Men and women who ate the most fruits and vegetables (8+ servings a day) were just as likely to develop cancer as those who ate the fewest fruits and vegetables, according to a 14-year study of nurses and doctors.

People who eat more fruits and vegetables do not live longer, according to study after study.

Some fruits and vegetables may have a higher probability of helping to prevent certain cancers.

For 22 years, researchers followed 90,476 premenopausal women. They discovered that people who consumed the most fruit during their teens (about 3 servings per day) had a

25% lower risk of breast cancer than those who consumed the least (0.5 servings a day). Those who ate a lot of apples, bananas, grapes, corn, and kale as children had a lower risk of breast cancer than women who ate a lot of oranges and kale. Fruit juices did not encourage younger participants to consume them in this trial.

2. Diabetes

Some research investigates whether certain fruits are associated with a higher risk of type 2 diabetes. While there hasn't been much research done on this subject yet, the preliminary findings are highly intriguing.

The study included more than 66,000 women from the Nurses' Health Study, 85,104 women from the Nurses' Health Study II, and 36,173 men from the Health Professionals Follow-up Study who did not have any serious chronic conditions. People who ate more whole fruits, particularly blueberries, grapes, and apples, had a lower chance of developing type 2 diabetes, according to the study. Another key discovery was that persons who consume more fruit juice had a higher risk of developing type 2 diabetes.

In addition, a study of more than 70,000 female nurses found that persons who ate a lot of green leafy vegetables and fruit had a lower risk of diabetes. Although the data isn't conclusive, women who consume fruit juice may be more likely to develop cancer.

This comes from a survey of over 2,300 men in Finland. Fruits and vegetables, particularly berries, may help to reduce the risk of type 2 diabetes.

3. Weight

Over a 24-year period, women and men who ate more fruits and vegetables than those who ate the same amount or cut back on their consumption were substantially more likely to lose weight in the Nurses' Health Study. Berries and apples, for example, are non-starchy fruits and vegetables that have been related to weight loss. People gained weight when they ate starchy foods such as potatoes, corn, and peas. Don't just increase your fruit and vegetable intake if you want to lose weight. Something else, such as white bread and crackers, must be eliminated first.

4. The health of a person's intestines

Indigestible fibre is found in fruits and vegetables, and it absorbs water and expands as it passes through the digestive system. This can assist if your bowels are irritated. Constipation can be relieved or avoided by forcing you to use the restroom regularly. Diverticulosis is less common in those who consume a lot of insoluble fiber, which makes meals more bulky and soft.

5. Vision

Eating a lot of fruits and vegetables might also help to keep your eyes healthy. This may help you avoid cataracts and macular degeneration, two prevalent aging-related eye illnesses that impact millions of people in their 60s and 70s each year. Cataract risk appears to be reduced by these two vitamins.

IN ALFAFA, ARE RICH IN SPROUTS

Why are they so good: One cup of alfalfa sprouts has less than 10 calories, is nearly fat-free, and contains saponins, which may aid in cancer prevention and cholesterol reduction.

The crunch of fresh, earthy vegetables: To savor their flavor and aroma, toss them into salads or on top of a lean turkey or veggie burger.

Alfalfa sprouts may be beneficial to persons who want to supplement their diet with more nutrients. They could also be low in calories and delicious. These seedlings may, among other things, help people lose weight, battle diabetes, enhance digestion, build bone health, and lower cholesterol levels. Many people believe that alfalfa sprouts are a rich source of plant estrogen, which is good for women's health, may help relieve the pain of menopause, and can regulate menstrual cycles.

Is it possible to buy alfalfa sprouts in a store?

Alfalfa sprouts are seedlings of the Medicago sativa plant, also known as alfalfa. They're still in their early twenties. If the bitterness of the plant's leaves bothers you, you can consume the young seedlings, which have a milder flavor and are high in nutrients, minerals, and antioxidants. Al-fal-fa, which means "father of all foods" and is native to Central Asia and areas of the Middle East, was given this name by the Arabs due to its powerful properties.

Alfalfa sprouts go well in salads, sandwiches, soups, and other savory foods. Some foods can also be served with them as a garnish. Alfalfa sprouts are still popular in Asian cultures, and you can make them at home.

Alfalfa sprouts nutritional information

Alfalfa sprouts may be high in minerals, vitamins C and A, and B vitamins like thiamin, riboflavin, and pantothenic acid. They may also be beneficial to your health due to their high mineral content. One cup of alfalfa sprouts (33g) has nearly 13% of your daily vitamin K requirements while only containing 7.6 calories and having a low glycemic index. For a low-calorie dish, that's a lot of vitamin K.

With roughly 2 grams of fiber in every 100 grams of sprouts, you can get a lot of fiber.

These nutrient-dense sprouts also have a lot of protein in them. Almost 8% of your daily protein requirements are found in 100 grams. Furthermore, the sprouts contain a large number of beneficial plant chemicals including as saponins and flavonoids. These substances can aid in the prevention and treatment of disease in your body.

Alfalfa sprouts offer a variety of beneficial properties, including the following:

1. It may aid in the battle against cancer

Phytoestrogens in sprouted sprouts help balance hormones and minimize inflammation. Sprouts also aid in the prevention of the formation of malignant cells by inhibiting the creation of new blood cells.

This medicine may be able to aid with Menopause and Menstrual abnormalities in women who take it.

Alfalfa sprouts are good for women because they contain a lot of vitamin K and phytoestrogens, which can help balance estrogen levels and alleviate menopause symptoms like mood swings. Vitamin K can help your blood clot, which is why it can help you stop bleeding.

2. It has the potential to assist you in shedding pounds

These sprouts are the perfect fiber-rich snack to keep you feeling full without adding a lot of calories to your diet because they just have a few calories. Additionally, the vitamins in these sprouts can assist to speed up the metabolism, increasing energy levels and boosting energy metabolism, making it simpler to burn fat while sleeping. Although eating too many alfalfa sprouts can be hazardous, including them in your salads every day can help you stay full.

3. It can aid in the treatment of type 2 diabetes

Alfalfa sprouts are high in fiber, making them a healthy option for diabetics. Alfalfa leaf powder extract decreases blood sugar levels in diabetics, according to an animal study published in the Polytechnic Journal. It's a good idea to do this because it helps manage diabetes and lowers the odds of it occurring in the first place. Sprout eaters are less prone to develop metabolic syndrome or other diabetes-related disorders.

4. Cholesterol levels could be reduced

Over the last 40 years, a lot of studies has been done to prove that alfalfa sprouts can help decrease cholesterol. This indicates that these foods are suitable for persons at risk of coronary heart disease. Lowering your LDL cholesterol levels is preferable to preventing plaque build-up in your arteries and blood vessels, which can reduce your risk of heart attacks and strokes.

5. It may aid in the battle against illnesses in your body

Alfalfa sprouts provide about 15% of your daily vitamin C requirements, making them an excellent immune system booster. Alfalfa sprouts may aid in the production of white blood cells, which can aid in the fight against infections and inflammation. Because vitamin C is so crucial in the collagen-making process, they also help with growth and repair.

6. It Might Assist With Food Digestibility

Dietary fiber aids digestion and aids in the passage of stool through the intestines. Alfalfa sprouts are high in fiber and can aid people who are suffering from constipation, diarrhoea, or other gastrointestinal issues.

7. It Has the Potential to Assist You in Growing and Restoring Yourself

Alfalfa sprouts have a high protein content. A single 100-gram meal provides nearly 10% of your daily protein requirements. This can help with muscle gain and fat loss, as well as growth, development, and repair throughout the body.

8. It has the potential to hasten the healing process

Alfalfa sprouts include vitamin K, which helps help the body's blood clotting. This can aid wound healing and lower infection risk. While too much vitamin K can lead to heart disease and blood clots, alfalfa sprouts in moderation should not cause these issues.

9. It is possible to avoid osteoporosis

To create strong bones, alfalfa sprouts are a wonderful source of magnesium, iron, calcium, and vitamin K. These sprouts aid in the prevention of osteoporosis by reducing the likelihood of it developing early.

10. It Has the Potential to Increase Fat Burning

These sprouts contain a variety of B vitamins, which can aid in the smooth functioning of the body's enzymatic reactions, hormone generation, energy metabolism, and other vital activities. When you don't receive enough B vitamins, a lot of negative things happen, and these sprouts can help you avoid a lot of them.

11. It aids in the care of one's skin

These alfalfa sprouts are strong in antioxidants and have been connected to anti-aging effects such as reducing wrinkles and blemishes, as well as boosting skin elasticity, so they could be beneficial to you. Antioxidants can make your skin look healthier as long as you consume them in moderation.

WHY APPLES, EXACTLY

Apples are the best source of pectin in the fruit, which has been shown to improve blood pressure, lower cholesterol, cut the incidence of colon and breast cancer, and may also aid with diabetes.

Using a few pieces, make your favorite sandwich. To make a quick and appetizing salad, combine them with field greens, toasted pecan halves, and a light dressing. You'll never run out of fresh ways to consume them because there are so many varieties.

Apples are the most popular fruit in the world, with over 7,000 different varieties.

A delicious red apple-like Red Delicious or a tart green apple will appeal to everyone. Everyone gets an apple.

They're commonly used in cooking to make pies, pastries, jam, and oatmeal, but they're also delicious on their own or with nut butter.

Apples are a very healthy fruit with many scientifically proven benefits, in addition to their versatility in the kitchen and vast range of colors and flavors.

Five reasons why apples are beneficial to your health

1. It is nutritious

Each bite of an apple is supposed to have a lot of nutrients.

People who consume 2,000 calories per day should have two cups of fruit per day, with a preference for whole fruits such as apples.

Apples are also high in polyphenols, which are a type of antioxidant that is beneficial to your health. Antioxidants are molecules that protect your cells from the dangerous compounds known as free radicals. These chemicals have the potential to induce cardiovascular disease and cancer.

These plant compounds are not listed on nutrition labels. Many of the health benefits of apples are presumably due to them.

Leave the skin on the apples if you want to get the most out of them. It has half the fiber and the majority of the polyphenols.

2. It's possible that it'll assist you in losing weight

Apples are high in fiber and water, making them feel filling.

Growing a sense of fullness is a great way to lose weight because it helps you control your hunger.

As a result, you may find yourself eating less energy.

According to one study, people who ate whole apples felt fuller for up to 4 hours longer than people who ate apple juice or purée.

Because entire apples slow down gastric emptying, the rate at which your stomach empties its contents, this happened.

Apple eaters may reduce their BMI, a weight-related risk factor for heart disease.

Polyphenols found in apples may also aid with weight loss.

3. It is beneficial to your cardiovascular system

People who consume a lot of apples have a lower risk of cardiovascular disease. One reason for this could be because they contain soluble fiber. People that eat much of this fiber have a lower cholesterol level.

Another reason may be that they are beneficial to your health because they contain polyphenols. Some, such as the flavonoid epicatechin, may help decrease blood pressure, according to the researchers.

According to studies, people who eat a lot of flavonoids had a lower risk of stroke.

They can also help you maintain a healthy blood pressure, protect your LDL cholesterol, and prevent plaque buildup in your arteries.

People who consume white-fleshed fruits and vegetables, such as apples and pears, had a lower chance of suffering a heart attack or stroke, according to another study. The risk of suffering a stroke was reduced by 9% for every 1/5 cup (25 grams) of apple slices consumed daily.

4. It has been related to a lower diabetes risk

Apples may help prevent type 2 diabetes as well. According to a collection of research, people who ate apples and pears had an 18% lower risk of developing type 2 diabetes. There is only one of these.

They contain a high amount of the antioxidant polyphenols quercetin and phloridzin, which may explain why they are beneficial.

Insulin resistance, which is a major risk factor for diabetes, may benefit from the anti-inflammatory characteristics of quercetin.

Phloridzin, on the other hand, is thought to reduce sugar absorption in the intestines, hence lowering blood sugar levels and minimizing the risk of diabetes.

5. It may aid in the maintenance of a healthy digestive system

Pectin, a type of fiber found in apples, is beneficial to your health. This implies it nourishes your gut's beneficial microorganisms.

Your gut microbiota affects your general health in a variety of ways, both good and bad. Gut health is often linked to overall health.

Because fiber cannot be broken down, it reaches your colon undamaged, encouraging the growth of beneficial microorganisms. Many people claim that it improves the

Bacteriodetes to Firmicutes ratio in the intestines.

Apples may be able to help you avoid obesity, type 2 diabetes, heart disease, and cancer by improving your gut bacteria.

THERE IS SOMETHING ABOUT AVOCADOS

Half a medium avocado has more than 4 grams of fiber and 15% of your daily folate requirements. Avocados are also high in monounsaturated fats and potassium, both of which are beneficial to your heart.

How to have fun with them: Avocados can be used to make a creamy sandwich spread or to add a few chunks to your favorite salsa to enhance the flavor of grilled chicken or fish.

Avocados are commonly thought to be healthy, but they may also aid digestion, reduce the risk of depression, and protect against cancer.

Academia is a berry that grows in the United States. They're also known as butter fruit or alligator pear. They thrive in warm climates.

Avocados are high in monounsaturated fatty acids and vitamins and minerals. You can gain a lot of benefits from them when you combine them with a healthy, varied diet.

Continue reading to learn more about how avocados can benefit your health and what to watch out for if you consume too many of them.

1. A large number of nutrients

Avocados are high in vitamin B6, as well as vitamins C and E. They also include magnesium and potassium. Lutein, beta carotene, and omega-3 fatty acids are also found in them.

Avocados are high in good, healthful fats, which can help people feel satisfied between meals. If you eat fat, which inhibits the digestion of carbohydrates, you can keep your blood sugar levels steady.

Every cell in the body requires fat. Eating healthy fats is beneficial to your skin, your body's ability to absorb fat-soluble vitamins, minerals, and other nutrients, and even your immune system.

2. Good for the heart

Every 100 grams of avocado has 76 milligrams of beta-sitosterol. Plants provide this natural plant sterol. Many people believe that consuming beta-sitosterol and other plant sterols daily will help them maintain optimal cholesterol levels, which is beneficial to their cardiovascular health.

3. Excellent for observing

Avocados include lutein and zeaxanthin, which are two compounds present in eye tissue. They defend against free radicals, which can cause harm, such as those produced by the sun.

Avocados' monounsaturated fatty acids also aid in the absorption of other beneficial fat-soluble antioxidants, such as beta carotene. As a result, eating avocados may reduce the risk of age-related macular degeneration.

4. It may help prevent osteoporosis

Half an avocado contains around 18% of the daily intake of vitamin K.

Many people overlook this nutrient, although it is critical for bone health. Getting adequate vitamin K can improve bone health by boosting calcium absorption and reducing calcium loss.

5. Components may be able to halt the progression of cancer

Avocado eaters do not have a lower cancer risk. Avocados, on the other hand, contain chemicals that may aid in the prevention of cancer.

Folate deficiency has been related to a lower risk of colon, stomach, pancreatic, and cervical malignancies, according to research. We don't understand how this association works, though. Half an avocado has about 59 micrograms of folate, which is 15% of the daily recommended amount.

Avocados are high in phytochemicals and carotenoids, both of which may help to prevent cancer. Cancer growth has been demonstrated to be slowed by carotenoids in particular.

A study published in 2013 looked into the potential health advantages of avocados for breast, oral, and throat malignancies. Most of the time, however, these links are made in laboratories rather than in controlled human studies. To be certain that these links exist, more research is needed.

BEET MAGIC

What makes beets so special? They're high in antioxidants, and they've been linked to reduced risk of cancer, heart disease, and inflammation. Beets are popular because they are naturally sweet and high in fiber and vitamin C, both of which are beneficial to one's health.

If you want to consume them, finely shred them and add to salads, or roast them with sweet potatoes and parsnips for a colorful and delectable side dish. Keep in mind that some cooking methods (such as boiling) will deplete the nutritional value of the vegetables. Remember to include the leafy green tops, which are high in iron and folate and can be prepared similarly to Swiss chard and spinach.

Beets are referred to as "beets" by many people. Beets are a colorful and adaptable vegetables. Their flavor and aroma are earthy.

Beets are also high in vitamins, minerals, and plant compounds, many of which have therapeutic benefits. They also give your dish a vibrant appearance.

Beets are also delicious and simple to incorporate into your diet, as they can be found in hummus, fries, salads, and other foods.

Here are several tempting ways to eat more beets, as well as five research-backed advantages of beets

1. Beet contains a high amount of nutrients while having a low-calorie count

Beets are packed with vitamins and minerals.

They offer a lot of vitamins and minerals that are necessary to your health, despite the fact that they are low in calories. They include a little amount of nearly every vitamin and mineral your body requires to stay healthy.

Beets are high in folate, a nutrient that is important for heart health, growth, and development.

They're also high in manganese, which helps with bone growth, nutrient metabolism, and brain function, among other things. Copper is also abundant, which is required for energy generation and the creation of some neurotransmitters.

This could be beneficial if you maintain healthy blood pressure.

2. They can aid in the reduction of excessive blood pressure, which is a major cause of heart disease

Beetroot juice drinkers may be able to significantly drop their systolic and diastolic blood pressure.

The pressure in your heart as it pumps, known as systolic blood pressure, appears to have a greater impact than the pressure in your heart when it relaxes, known as diastolic blood pressure. Raw beets, on the other hand, may have a greater impact than cooked beets.

It could be due to the high nitrate content of this root vegetable. When food nitrates are broken down, the body produces nitric oxide, which reduces blood pressure.

Beets are also high in folate, which can aid in blood pressure reduction. Despite conflicting evidence, several studies suggest that consuming extra folate may help decrease blood pressure.

Bear in mind, however, that the effect of beets on blood pressure is just temporary. As a result, you'll need to consume them on a regular basis to observe results.

3. It can assist you in improving your athletic abilities

Several studies have suggested that consuming nitrates, such as those found in beets, can help athletes perform better.

Nitrates may boost your physical performance by increasing the efficiency of your mitochondria, which are the energy-producing sections of your cells.

Beetroot juice, according to one study, can promote endurance by making it take longer to get tired, improving cardiorespiratory function, and making athletes more efficient.

Beet juice, on the other hand, has been demonstrated to boost cycling performance and oxygen consumption by up to 20 per cent.

It's crucial to understand that eating beets or drinking their juice raises blood nitrate levels immediately. This is why, to get the most out of them, you should have them a few hours before you head to the gym or compete.

4. It has anti-inflammatory properties

Beets contain anti-inflammatory pigments called betalain.

Chronic inflammation has been related to obesity, heart disease, liver disease, and cancer, so this could help with a variety of different aspects of your health.

A study of 24 persons with high blood pressure found that drinking 8.5 ounces (250 mL) of beet juice for two weeks reduced CRP and tumor necrosis factor-alpha levels (TNF-a).

Consuming pills containing beetroot extract also helped those with osteoarthritis, a disorder that causes inflammation in the joints, feel less pain and discomfort.

Beetroot juice and extract have also been discovered to aid rats that have been injected with hazardous, injury-causing substances to lessen inflammation.

Still, a further human study is needed to discover if eating beets in moderation as part of a healthy diet has the same anti-inflammatory effects. This is why more research is needed.

5. May improve the health of your stomach

One cup of beets has 3.4 grams of fiber, making them a good source of fiber.

Fiber isn't broken down by the body and goes straight to the colon, where it feeds good bacteria and makes stools bulkier.

This can improve your digestive health, make you more regular, and help you avoid problems like constipation, inflammatory bowel disease (IBS), and diverticulitis.

Fiber, on the other hand, has been linked to a lower risk of chronic diseases like colon cancer, heart disease, and type 2 diabetes, among other things.

WHAT IS THE PURPOSE OF HEALTHY EATING?

A good diet provides several health benefits, including strengthening bones, protecting the heart, preventing disease, and increasing mood.

Lean proteins, whole grains, healthy fats, and a rainbow of fruits and vegetables are among the healthiest foods available.

Furthermore, eating healthy entails substituting more nutritious foods for those containing trans fats, extra salt, or sugar. Let's talk about why eating healthy and why.

1. The likelihood of developing cancer is reduced

Antioxidant-rich diets can reduce cancer risk by preventing cell damage.

Cancer is more prone to occur when there are more free radicals in the body. Antioxidants can aid in the removal of these substances, reducing the likelihood of them occurring.

Antioxidants can be obtained from phytochemicals present in fruits and vegetables by people who consume a lot of them. Phytochemicals are the antioxidants in question. Some of the most prevalent phytochemical antioxidants are beta-carotene, vitamin C, and vitamin E.

Even while human trials aren't clear, lab and animal research reveals that particular antioxidants help reduce free radical damage caused by cancer, according to a report published by the National Cancer Institute.

Obese people are more likely to develop cancer and suffer a worse prognosis. These hazards could be reduced by maintaining a healthy weight.

In 2014, those who consumed a lot of fruits were less likely to get malignancies of the upper gastrointestinal tract.

Colorectal cancer is reduced by eating a diet rich in vegetables, fruits, and fiber, while liver cancer is reduced by eating a diet rich in fiber.

2. It has the potential to lift your spirits.

Diet and mood are linked, according to some research

Researchers discovered in 2016 that high-glycemic-load meals can cause people to become unhappy and weary.

Refined carbs, such as those found in soft drinks, cakes, white bread, and biscuits, are abundant in a high glycemic load diet. Glycemic load is lower in vegetables, whole fruit, and whole grains, which implies they contain less sugar.

If you suspect you might be depressed, see a doctor or a mental health expert.

3. Improving the health of one's intestines

The colon is home to numerous natural bacteria. They're involved in everything from metabolism to digesting.

Vitamins K and B are produced by some bacteria strains, which are beneficial to the colon. These bacteria and viruses are likewise fought by these strains.

Your gut microbiome changes when you don't consume enough fiber and eat a lot of sweets and fat. This results in inflammation in the affected area.

However, eating a variety of vegetables, fruits, legumes, and whole grains provides a mix of prebiotics and probiotics, which aid in the growth of beneficial bacteria in your colon.

Fiber is a type of prebiotic found in beans, grains, fruits, and vegetables. It also aids in regular bowel motions, which can help prevent colon cancer and diverticulitis.

4. The ability to remember information has improved

A balanced diet can help your brain and cognition stay in good shape.

A 2015 study discovered nutrients and meals that help protect against cognitive decline and dementia.

5. Preventing Weight Loss

Maintaining a healthy weight can reduce the risk of developing long-term health issues. Obese or overweight people are more likely to develop a variety of ailments, including heart disease.

Many healthy foods, such as fruits, vegetables, and legumes, have fewer calories than processed foods.

The Dietary Guidelines for Americans 2015–2020 can help people determine how many calories they need to consume.

Maintaining a healthy, low-processed-food diet can help a person stay below their daily calorie restriction without having to keep track of what they eat.

Fiber in your diet is critical for weight management. Dietary fiber is abundant in plant-based foods, which helps people feel fuller for longer periods.

CONCLUSION

It's not by chance that you're in good health. It requires that you work for it, a healthy lifestyle, and the occasional checkup and test are all necessary.

Fibre, whole grains, fresh fruits and vegetables, "good" or unsaturated fats, and omega-3 fatty acids are all important components of a balanced diet. Inflammation can harm tissue, joints, artery walls, and organs, hence these dietary components help to reduce it. Another component of healthy eating is limiting processed foods. Sugar-sweetened beverages, sweets, and foods produced with highly refined grains can cause blood sugar increases, which can contribute to hunger. Diabetes, obesity, heart disease, and even dementia are all linked to high blood sugar.

www.ingramcontent.com/pod-product-compliance
Lightning Source LLC
Chambersburg PA
CBHW060214260726
48658CB00005BA/2030